Beauty Secrets for Women 35 and Older

How to Look Younger and be the Most Beautiful Version of Yourself

Jane Moore

Table of Contents

Contents

Introduction – Beauty at Any Age

As woman, we tend not to like to think about aging. We falsely believe that as we age our beauty is going to diminish, yet nothing could be further from the truth. Looking good and feeling your best is only a few chapters away.

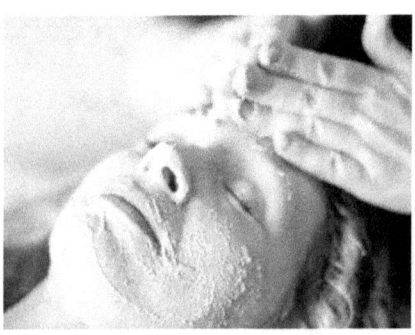

You can learn how to age beautifully and to enjoy the years that are ahead of you. In fact, don't be surprised if you look better now than you did when you were younger. It happens often.

We will give you natural healthy options and we will talk about things you should avoid to help you look your best. Following are timeless principles that will never die – you can use them today, tomorrow, and ten years from now. They are effective whether you're 35+ or 65+. But remember what you do to maintain your beauty today will be reflected when you are older too!

So how did they manage aging beautifully? It certainly is something most of us struggle with every day. Aging is a billion dollar industry today. Honestly many of the skin care products we buy to help us look our best, do not work, and in some cases it actually poses a health risk. So instead let's look at healthy ways to stay beautiful today and into the future.

We will look at both the external you and the internal you, because your internal well being is reflected on your external being. By the time you are through this book, you will have all the tools you need to look your best – to let your beauty shine.

Are you ready? Let's get started.

Beauty Secret #1 Know Your Skin Type

In order for you to give your skin what it needs most, you need to know what type of skin type you have. If someone has told you your skin type before, the best thing you can do is forget what you learned.

Typically, you would hear the categories, dry, oily and combination skin. The trouble is that there are a host of other problems that can affect your skin type like sun damage, acne, eczema, or rosacea to name just a few. In addition, you can have more than one skin type. You might be oily and sensitive or dry, but blemish prone, you might have combination skin and sun damage.

The likelihood of combination skin increases as you get older. Let's have a look at your skin type and get into it a little more so that you can do a better job of keeping your skin glowing, healthy and more youthful.

What Influences Your Skin Type

There are tons of things that can influence your skin type both internally and externally. To do a good job of evaluating your skin you should consider these factors that can affect your skin. Consider which ones are affecting your skin.

- Climate
- Diet
- Genetic Predisposition
- Hormones
- Medications
- Pollution
- Skin Disorders
- Smoking
- Second-hand Smoke
- Stress
- Unprotected Sun Exposure
- Prolonged Sun Exposure
- Your Skin-Care Routine

Ingredients That Can Make Your Skin Worse

What many of us aren't aware of is that the use of certain products and ingredients can make your skin issues worth. For example, many products that are used to treat acne contain high amounts of alcohol or other irritating ingredient, which can cause your skin to become dry and irritated, which in turn can lead to additional oil production.

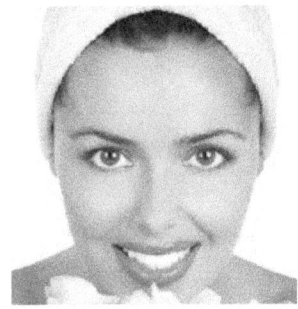

If you are using any products that contain irritating ingredients you won't know what your true skin type is, at least not until you stop their use.

If you use thick-textured products, often it can lead to clogged pores. If your skin cells don't exfoliate properly, your skin will look dull and old. It can even cause wrinkles. In order to know what's going on with your skin you have to know if your products are to blame.

Ingredients that can affect your skin care products include:

- Abrasive Scrubbing Agents
- Alcohol
- Fragrances from essential oils
- Harsh Cleansing Agents
- Drying Cleansing Agents
- Irritants
- Menthol

- Pore-Clogging Waxes
- Thick Emollients

Identify Your True Skin Type

Once you have ruled out any factors, including ingredients that can be problematic you are much closer to determining your true skin type. At some point most of us deal with combination skin. That's because the center of your face has more oil glands than there are more pores to get clogged along the 'T Zone.' In addition, areas around your nose and eyes tend to be more sensitive.

Knowing your skin type helps you to choose the right kinds of products and the right skin routines.

From here, we will start to look at beauty secrets you can put to work in your life. Let's get started.

Beauty Secret #2 – Choose the Right Skin Care Products

Women desire to have beautiful glowing skin. Actually, these days' men also work hard to keep their skin looking its best. It has been proven that we are hardwired to be attracted to people with a glowing complexion and clear skin. We do it and our ancestors did it. Why is that? It's because this represents good health and in ancient time this would actually translate to longevity.

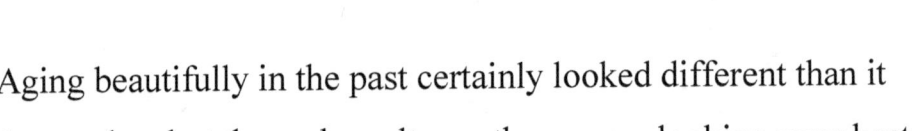

Aging beautifully in the past certainly looked different than it does today, but the end result was the same – looking your best and aging beautifully.

Let's get started looking at the various types of skin care that are available to you. These are healthy options that can keep you as beautiful today as you were yesterday.

Shea Butter Skin Care

Often Shea Butter is referred to as Karite. Shea Butter comes from the Shea Nut Tree, which is found in the western region of

Africa. The Shea Nut Tree fruit has a nut inside it. This nut is crushed, dried, and then ground. The powder is then boiled so t which allows a green substance to be released. This substance rises to the top and when it solidifies, you have what we call Shea Butter, which is a very popular skin care treatment.

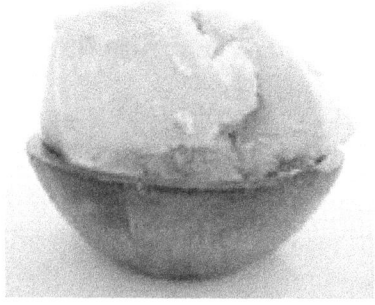

The use of Shea Butter isn't new. For centuries, African women have been moisturizing their skin and protecting it from the sun and wind using Shea Butter.

Shea butter has some unique qualities. It is these qualities that give it so beneficial to the skin. It is high in fat, Vitamin E, Vitamin A and Vitamin F. All of these help to enhance cell generation and capillary circulation in your skin, while at the same time providing superior moisturizing.

You can see why Shea butter has been such a popular choice for so long. Shea Butter extraordinary qualities mean it is chosen to be an ingredient in many of the products we have available to us today. You can also buy pure Shea Butter. This is your best option, because if you choose products with other ingredients you are going to want to make sure that these other ingredients are natural and that the product is chemical free. Pure Shea Butter is really the best way to enjoy the benefits it has to offer.

Because of the moisturizing and emollient properties of Shea Butter it can penetrate the skin, which is something most products cannot do. You can use Shea butter as your daily moisturizer but it can also be used to treat dry skin, dermatitis, eczema, burns, dark spots and blemishes.

Wait – there's more - Shea Butter can be used to reduce wrinkles. In fact, many women report that Shea Butter is more effective than some of the most expensive creams on the market. It is also is a natural sunscreen with an equivalent of around an SPF 3 protection.

Research has shown that Shea Butter has medicinal qualities. Its anti-inflammatory qualities and because it contains stigma sterol which is the sterol that is referred to as "the anti-stiffness factor Shea Butter could prove helpful in treating arthritis.

Shea butter has a shelf life of approx. 24 months and you should always store it in a cool place. There is no known toxin associated with Shea Butter, which makes it an excellent choice in skin care.

Jojoba Skin Care

In the Sonora Desert, which is found in Arizona, you will find the Simmondsia Chinensis plant growing. This is where Jojoba comes from. It's also found growing throughout Mexico.

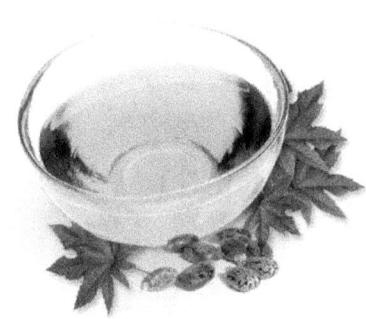

We know the benefits of Jojoba for skin care, but our ancestors used Jojoba for far more, including treating insect bites, burns, stretch marks and many other skin issues.

Jojoba oil isn't actually an oil – rather it is a botanical extract. It was back in the 1930's that it was discovered to be 98% pure liquid wax ester, which means it has similar properties to the sebum found in your skin. Sperm whale oil is the only other place this has been found. It is this wax ester that makes Jojoba so desirable.

Jojoba oil is easily absorbed so you don't have to worry about that annoying oily residue that some products have. If you use

Jojoba as your daily moisturizer you will enjoy youthful, silky, soft skin. It has even been an effective acne treatment. Be generous with your Jojoba and use it all over your body. It is also makes an excellent lip balm and make up remover.

If you already have wrinkles, not to worry, because studies have shown that when Jojoba oil is used continuously as a moisturizer, it can actually decrease fine lines and wrinkles by up to 26%.

Jojoba is of the most popular ingredients in the cosmetic industry, because it is considered to be high quality. It is used in all kinds of natural moisturizers, and you will also find it in numerous anti aging skin care products. Don't be surprised if you find Jojoba referred to as a 'miracle oil.'

Ayurvedic Skin Care

For more than 5000 years women (and some men) have been using Ayurvedic skin care, which is built around medicinal practices, philosophical and psychological practices.

The holistic approach of Ayurvedic skin treats all of you, not just your skin – your mind, body, and spirit will all be treated. Ayurvedic skin care has three basic principles called humors:

1. Vata
2. Pitta
3. Kapha

Each is derived from five natural elements, and it will reach deep into the body rather than just touching your skin's surface with some cream that you put on your face. With Ayurvedic you can keep your skin soft and radiant without spending a fortune.

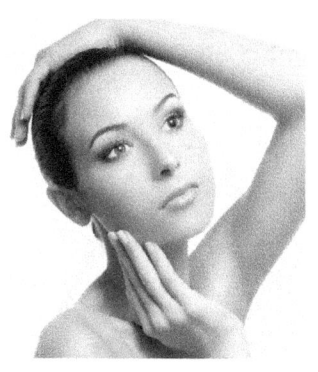

According to Ayurvedic, the accumulation of Vata in your body will cause your skin to become dry. Vata commonly occurs during the fall and winter months or in cold climates. You might be surprised to learn that your diet can disturb Vata.

When there is too much Vata in your body, your hair tends to be dry and dull, you have brittle nails and you have dry cracked skin. According to Ayurvedic skin care, the secret to aging beautifully is to keep your Vata healthy and balanced. Many of these tips are healthy on their own even if they were not associated to Ayurvedic Vata.

Eat Seeds and Nuts

Add nuts and seed to your diet and watch how it improves the condition of your skin. Eat healthy fats to balance your Vata.

Sip Your Tea

Since Vata is dry and for you to enjoy more youthful skin you need to counteract these qualities. Make sure you stay hydrated. A good way to do this is with warm herbal teas since not only will they hydrate you, they will also warm you.

Eat Plenty of Vegetables

Make sure you are eating lots of vegetables that have high water content as these are easier to digest. They include vegetables like cucumbers, carrots, lettuce, etc. These are Tri-Doshic vegetables, which means they contain Vata, Pita, and Kapha. This makes them perfect for your skin.

Exercise

Exercise stops the accumulation of cold Vata. Choose exercises that will provide you with energy rather than draining you.

These days we are far less active than our ancestors were and there is no question it has a negative effect on our overall health and your youthful vitality. In other words, if you aren't exercising, you are going to age faster.

Just Breathe

You've likely had someone tell you 'just breathe' when you are facing an insurmountable problem. When you are dealing with higher than normal levels of emotional stress it will aggravate Vata and it will suck your vital juices right out of your skin, which will cause you to become dehydrated and look old. Participate in Yogic breathing and meditation to reduce your stress.

How to do Yogic Breathing

1. Start by lying on your back
2. Place one palm on your belly, and the other on your chest.
3. Inhale deep into your belly and then inhale into your ribs to expand your rib cage.
4. Let the air completely fill your lungs.
5. Keep track of your breathing in and out.
6. Let the air move in the opposite order you inhale.

7. Repeat for 5-10 minutes to calm you.

Get Enough Sleep

If you aggravate your Vata you will become restless and then you will find you have problems sleeping properly. Insomnia sets in and your skin suffers as a result of it. You begin to age much faster.

Ayurvedic doctors say that if your desire is to have healthy, glowing, youthful skin you must get a minimum of seven hours sleep.

Honey Skin Care

Honey has long been used to treat wounds and as part of skin

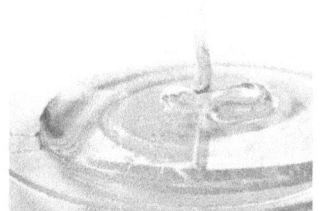

care. Honey is extremely powerful and it is a natural antioxidant and anti-microbial. Honey can protect your skin from the dangers of UV rays and it can rejuvenate the skin. It's why honey is so popular in natural beauty cosmetics.

Honey is humectants. This means it will draw and bind water in the air to your skin. If you want to give your skin an incredible treat, try a honey mask.

1. Apply honey evenly to your slightly damp skin.
2. Leave it on for anywhere from one hour.
3. Gently wash off with warm water.

This will hydrate and soften your skin. If your skin is super dry, feel free to use it daily.

Honey also makes an excellent cleanser. All you need is a drop of honey and mix it with water in the palm of your hand and then cleanse your face like you normally would and rinse.

Honey is an excellent choice for skin care that will help you maintain your youthfulness with healthy, glowing skin.

Aloe Vera Skin Care

Aloe has been used for many, many years - generation's back, to treat burns and wounds. It has self healing qualities, which means when the plant is torn it will automatically shrink the wound and create a watertight seal.

Aloe Vera is close to the PH of your skin so it works with any skin type. It will improve the fibroblast cells in your skin that which produce collagen and elastin. The more fiber your skin has, the more youthful you are going to look.

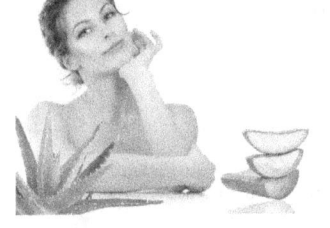

Aloe Vera can open your skin's pores so that they are able to do a better job of receiving nutrients. If your skin is dehydrated it is going to be dry and flaky and this can happen at any age. Aloe can help to prevent dehydration.

Aloe also has tons of antioxidants that fight free radicals, which are responsible for the aging of your skin.

Summary of Skin Care

That was easy, wasn't it? Each of these skin care ingredients can be found stand alone or in combination with other ingredients. Always read the labels carefully.

Now it's time to move on and help you learn how to determine your skin type. Are you ready?

Beauty Secret #2 Awareness

Today, many if not most, of all the skin care and beauty products on the market contain endocrine-disrupting chemicals and carcinogens that are linked with a number of cancers including breast cancer.

Our grandmothers and great grandmothers didn't face this dilemma. They relied on simple processes and natural ingredients to keep their skin looking beautiful, glowing and youthful. Don't believe me, just have a look at some of the pictures from past generations and notice the 'glow,' and they weren't dependent on a bunch of chemicals to create that glow.

If you want to make healthier choices, start by asking yourself which skin care and cosmetics you don't want to live without and what healthier substitutes you can use that have fewer chemicals in them.

The best way to shun chemicals is by using fewer commercial products, and opting for healthier natural beauty secrets. You might even decide to make some of your own products. This is a lot easier than you might think, and we will talk more about that later in the book.

Why Choose Natural Skin Care

There are many many benefits to using natural skin care products. With natural skin care you will actually enjoy softer, smoother and healthier skin than any chemical based product can offer. Using natural skin care products can actually postpone the aging process and in some cases reverse it.

Natural skin care is a far healthier choice and you do not have

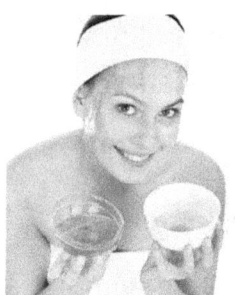 to worry about the many risks associated with chemical based products. Whenever you are purchasing skin care products you need to take the time to read the ingredients. You need to be careful since the labels don't always tell the full picture and they can be deceiving.

What you may not be aware of, is that the FDA doesn't regulate the chemicals used in skin care products. The beauty industry is for the most part it is unregulated. The ingredients may not be tested and the real effects may not be known.

Watch for empty natural claims and be careful of words like 'organic' or 'natural' and actually take the time to read the label.

In the US, for a product to have the USDA certified organic seal at least 95% of the ingredients must bet organic, but the problem is the other 5% of ingredients can be anything including chemical based.

There are all kinds of toxic chemicals floating around in skin care and cosmetics that pose a very real risk to you over the long term and ironically, many of these products actually cause your skin to age faster, not slower. Have you ever noticed that the woman in their 70s or 80s who used fewer chemical based products on their skin have younger looking skin. Don't believe me, do your own little survey.

You might believe that women who are the most diligent with their skin care regimes would age slower and maintain their beauty longer. However, it seems that those that use fewer products age slower. While there is no science to back this, the belief is that the chemicals cause faster aging. In addition there is the worry that many of these ingredients are linked to cancer.

No beauty regime that puts you at risk of developing cancer is worth it.

Read Labels for Synthetic Ingredients

Here's a rule that you can live by - If you can't pronounce the words listed on the ingredients then it is likely they are synthetic chemicals. Words such as DMDM or PEG should be a warning that these are chemicals and putting them on your skin isn't a good idea if you want to age beautifully.

G715742/2 - SKŁADNIKI / INGREDIENTS: • AQUA / WATER • CYCLOPENTASILOXANE • DIMETHICONE • GLYCERIN • POLYGLYCERYL-4 ISOSTEARATE • CETYL PEG/PPG-10/1 DIMETHICONE • HEXYL LAURATE • PENTYLENE GLYCOL • DISTEARDIMONIUM HECTORITE • METHYLPARABEN • CELLULOSE GUM • ALUMINUM HYDROXIDE • MAGNESIUM SULFATE • PHENOXYETHANOL • DISODIUM STEAROYL GLUTAMATE • TRISTEARIN • ACETYLATED GLYCOL STEARATE • ACRYLATES COPOLYMER • BUTYLPARABEN. [+/- MAY CONTAIN: • CI 77891 / TITANIUM DIOXIDE • CI 77492, CI 77499, CI 77491 / IRON OXIDES]   Code F.I.L. : B12815/2

Look for words you know, like Lavender, Aloe Vera, Aloe, Ylang, Vitamin A, Vitamin E, etc. – these you can rely on. If you can pronounce them and you recognize them they are going to have a positive effect on your beauty.

You should also avoid synthetic fragrances. There are hundreds of chemicals and toxic phthalates in a synthetic fragrance. I know this can be a hard one, especially if you have a favorite fragrance. The next best thing is to sprits' it onto your clothing rather than your body, but remember, you are still inhaling. In addition so many of those wonderfully smelling 'after bath' products are also contain synthetic fragrance.

It was actually easier for our ancestors to create a healthy, safe, effective beauty regime than it is for us. If you want to reduce your exposure to chemicals purchase natural beauty products or opt to make your own products using common household ingredients.

Products to Be Cautious About

There are many different ingredients that you should avoid because they pose health risks, which we will delve into in more detail later. Opt for healthier choices, and go natural. Here are some of the products to be careful of.

- Sunscreens that may contain estrogen mimicking chemicals.
- Skin lighteners containing hydroquinone
- Shaving creams, hair gels, hair spray and hair dyes that contain fungicides, nonylphenol, isobutene, etc.
- Nail polish and nail polish removers with formaldehyde, DBP, toluene, etc.

- Moisturizers, and skin creams that contain PAHs, petrolatum, etc.
- Liquid hand soaps containing triclosan or triclocarban
- Heavily scented products
- Anti-aging creams that contain BHA acids, lactic, glycolic, AHA acids, etc.

Summary

When you first saw 'Awareness' as your second beauty secret, you were likely puzzled, wondering what that has to do with looking beautiful and staying youthful. Now you know! You are your own best advocate for making sure that you are giving your body what it needs to age beautifully. Remember, your skin is your largest organ.

By being aware about the decisions you make for the products you use you can make 'wise' choices and ensure you provide your body only with safe choices, which in turn will help you age gracefully and stay youthful.

Beauty Secret #3 – Watch for Chemicals

Your skin can't filter out the toxins and impurities from skin care products and cosmetics that have chemicals in them. Natural skin care doesn't have these toxins that your body has to deal with. They are gentler and they nourish the skin.

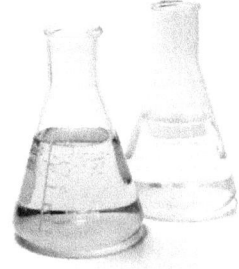 The Oxford Dictionary defines natural as, *"existing in, or caused by nature; not artificial; uncultivated; wild existing in natural state; not disguised or altered."* This definition seems pretty straight forward, yet the skin care industry has managed to stretch the meaning of the word 'natural' in their products so that it doesn't resemble natural in any way.

When you are looking at buying a product, start by having a look at the label. It's pretty common to see a long list of chemical names, followed by the words "derived from natural substances." If you are like most people, you think this refers to real natural ingredients, but in fact it does not – it's terribly misleading and far too often misunderstood. Of course, that's the goal of the product manufacturer.

Let's look at an example. "Sodium Hydroxysultaine" is a common ingredient and often it is followed by the words "derived from coconut oil." That leads consumers to think that this is derived from natural coconut. Very rarely this is the case – it is derived from natural coconut oil, but even in those rare occasions a chemical solvent is used to extract the natural ingredient. In the majority of cases, there is no natural coconut oil even used.

Beauty Tip #4 - Organic Skin Care

Organic is not the same as natural. The Oxford dictionary defines organic as, *"produced and involving production without the use of pesticides, artificial fertilizers or synthetic chemicals."*

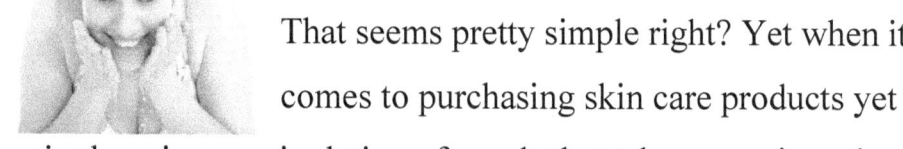

That seems pretty simple right? Yet when it comes to purchasing skin care products yet again there is a manipulation of words that takes organic and natural completely out of context.

For example, let's look at shampoo. Almost all shampoo has the ingredient Cocamide DEA listed, which is the foaming agent. DEA contains Diethanolamine, which is a known carcinogen. This means the product is no longer natural or safe.

When a label reads organic, you think it has no chemicals and that's exactly what they want you to think. These companies use the chemistry definition of organic, which reads *"a compound that contains a carbon atom."* This leads to a lot of confusion and misguided decisions, because how would you know that.

Let's look at an example. Let's say a company uses "Methyl Paraben," which is a toxic petrochemical preservative. Believe it or not, they will actually call it organic and they do this because it comes from leaves that have rotted over thousands of years, eventually turning into crude oil, which is then used to make the preservative. When you see the word organic you think pure and good and that's not always so.

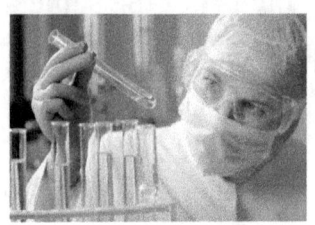

Another problem is that many manufacturers claim to use organic herbs in their products. However, with those organic herbs often come other ingredients that are derived from chemicals and unsafe.

There are no regulations on using the term organic unless it is for 'certified organic.' Only with "certified organic" can you be sure it is authentic.

Beauty Tip #5 - Humectants

Humectants are commonly found in skin care products. When you apply a cream, it should keep your skin moist. Many creams accomplish this using a film that suffocates the skin, stopping the loss of moisture from your skin. This is accomplished with humectants.

Natural humectants like glycerin pull water from the surrounding air and pull it to your skin keeping your skin moist. They depend on moisture in the air. If you live in a dry climate the moisture will actually be drawn away from your skin.

Three popular humectants are elastin, collagen and keratin, which usually come from animals. Some skin care companies have been busy making claims that special animal proteins are used to replace aging cells, but there is no science to back this claim up. These molecules can't penetrate your skin because they are too large, and even if they could be broken down your immune system would reject them as a foreign object.

Lecithin is an excellent humectants that provides natural phospholipids, which attract water from the surrounding air and then hold the water in areas of your skin that require moisture without creating a barrier level.

We live in an environment that strips away the natural phospholipids on our skin. This includes the wind, sun, pollution, detergents, and skin cleansers. The result is rough skin.

The only job of your top layer of skin is to provide a protective barrier. It does not metabolize the phospholipids that are in your top layer of the skin. A current study confirmed that when you topically apply plant phospholipids it will restore the skin's barrier function and protect against harmful substances.

3 Natural Humectants to Look For

Look for these three healthier choices that will actually work better than their chemical counterparts do.

1. **Glycerin** - The main use of glycerin is as a moisturizer for dry, rough skin. A number of studies have shown glycerin to have strong humectant properties that draw water to your skin's outer layer.

2. **Lecithin -** This natural moisturizer is made from soybeans, and it is able to penetrate the epidermis to reach the cellular level.

3. **Panthenol -** Panthenol or B5 is a natural anti-inflammatory and it has anti itching qualities. The skin is able to easily absorb panthenol and it is a highly effective acne treatment.

3 Synthetic Humectants to Avoid

Synthetic humectants are made from chemicals that are associated with a number of side effects ranging from mild to very serious.

1. **Propylene Glycol** – Causes irritation and contact dermatitis

2. **PEG compounds** (i.e. Polyethylene Glycol) – may contain the toxic by-product dioxane

3. **Ethylene/Diethylene Glycol** – Causes irritation and contact dermatitis

Humectants are a key ingredient in your skin care. Choose healthy!

Beauty Tip #6 - Emollients

Emollients protect your skin by creating a barrier and preventing dryness. Water is the best emollient, but water evaporates quickly its effects are minimal. Emollient oils are used to hold the water to your skin.

Synthetic emollients coat your skin much like if you wrapped your skin with plastic wrap. It does not breathe and this can cause your skin to become irritated. Even more of a concern is that research has shown that some of the synthetic emollients accumulate in the lymph nodes and the liver.

Natural emollients are a much better choice, because they will nourish your skin. The enzymes of your skin will metabolize natural emollients and absorbed them.

4 Natural Emollients to Look For

Look for these powerful natural emollients.

1. **Avocado** – Proves a natural way to nurture your skin that is chemical free. The oil of avocado is found in many

quality beauty products. Avocado contains essential nutrients that moisturize and soothe your skin. They help you age beautifully, reducing fine lines and wrinkles.

2. **Rosehip** – It is found in numerous skin care products especially in products that reduce wrinkles. Rosehip oil has many anti aging qualities and it will give you a youthful glow.

3. **Shea Butter** – Extracted from the kernels of the Shea nut, this oil is soothing to dry skin.

4. **Jojoba Butter** – Is an excellent skin moisturizer that is very similar to the human sebum, so it is able to protect the skin. It is very valuable in slowing the aging process.

4 Synthetic Emollients to Avoid

Synthetic emollients are made from chemicals and can be found in many skin care products. Here are some of the most common synthetic emollients you should avoid.

1. **Synthetic alcohols** – Any of these ingredients Benzyl, Butyl, Cetearyl, Cetyl, Glyceryl, Isopropyl, Myristyl propyl, or Propylene.

2. **PEG compounds** – It often contains the toxic by-product dioxane such as PEG- 45 Almond Glyceride.

3. **Hydrocarbons** - Contains carcinogens and mutagenic Polycyclic Aromatic Hydrocarbons (PAHs).

4. **Silicone Oils** - This is like putting a plastic wrap on your skin. It is reported to cause tumors on test animals. They include chemicals like dimethicone, cyclomethycaine, or copolyol.

Beauty Tip # 7 - Emulsifiers

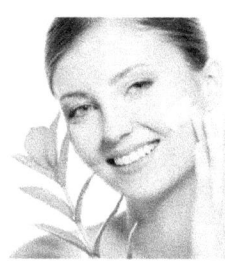

Emulsifiers are used to hold ingredients together that would normally would not mix. You often see emulsifiers in products that require you to shake them. Synthetic emulsifiers are usually petroleum based. Natural emulsifiers come from various nuts and berries so they are a much healthier choice.

4 Natural Emulsifiers to Look For

Rather than choosing the popular chemical emulsifiers, we encourage you to think like your caveman ancestors for these natural emulsifier options. They are healthy and do not have the dangers associated with chemicals.

1. **Jojoba** - – It's an excellent skin moisturizer that is very similar to the human sebum, so it protects your skin. It isn't oily or greasy.
2. **Candelilla** – This wax is effective in treating skin inflammation and skin allergies.
3. **Rice Bran** –It is a small molecule so it can easily penetrate the skin.

4. **Quince Seed** – It's one of the oldest cultivated herbs around. It's rich in vitamins and minerals, has superior moisture retaining and the benefits of skin rejuvenation.

4 Synthetic Emulsifiers to Avoid

Synthetic emulsifiers are based on harmful chemicals. Here are four of the most common synthetic emulsifiers to avoid

1. Laurate, Isopropyl Stearate, Palmitate, Oleate, etc.
2. PEG Compounds (may contain the toxin dioxane)
3. Alkoxylated Amides (can turn into carcinogens in the body)
4. Silicone, Ozokerite, Ceresin, and Montan Waxes

Beauty Tip # 8 - Surfactants

Surfactants work on your skin's surface dissolving the oils that trap dirt in and allowing them to be washed away. This is why they are added to skin cleansers. The problem is that these surfactants usually contain the carcinogen dioxin.

If you still don't want to believe there are dangers with this carcinogen, consider this - this same carcinogen was sprayed during Agent Orange in the Vietnam jungle. This resulted in thousands of birth defects in Vietnam and an increase in cancer rates for US and Australian military personnel that sprayed the agent.

4 Natural Surfactants to Look For

A far safer choice is natural foaming agents that cleanse your skin and hair without removing natural oils, and you won't have to worry that they might make you really sick or even kill you. They won't age your skin and you will age beautifully.

1. **Yucca Extract** – Yucca is used to heal the skin. In shampoo, it adds volume and shine. The high saponin gives it its soapy texture.

2. **Soapwort** - Externally it is used to cure *skin* problems like psoriasis, eczema, acne, boils, etc. This herb is rich in saponins, nature's cleansing.

3. **Quillaja Bark Extract** – Acting as a foaming agent it is a superior option over synthetic surfactant.

4. **Castile Soap** – It is made from 100% olive oil. It is gentle and it is very good for your skin. It also contains Squalene, which helps your skin to retain moisture.

6 Synthetic Surfactants to Avoid

These foaming agents make you feel like your skin care is working great, but actually what it's doing is putting your health at risk. Avoid the following synthetic surfactants.

1. PEG (Polyethylene Glycol) compounds
2. Dioctyl Sulfosuccinate
3. DEA compounds
4. Any ingredient that has Sulphate in the name
5. Any ingredient that has Sodium in the name
6. Any ingredient that has Lauryl in the name

There are others, but these are the main ones.

Beauty Tip # 9 - Preservatives

It is natural for decay to occur in skin care products. They aren't designed to last indefinitely. Skin care and cosmetics that use natural ingredients should have a limited shelf life.

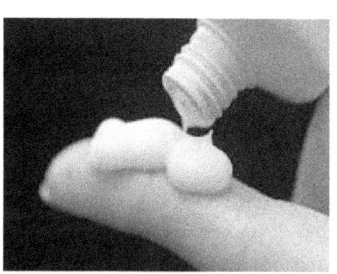

On the other hand, synthetic chemical preservatives are effective at preserving products for extended periods of time, but their safety has not been proven.

You should give serious thought to using products that contain these chemicals. It's much wiser to avoid synthetic preservatives and instead seek out products that are natural – these will help you age gracefully and beautifully.

4 Natural Preservatives to Look For

1. **Vitamin E** – It is more than a preservative, because it has very good healing and antioxidant properties.
2. **Thyme Essential Oil** - It is an excellent preservative thanks to the anti fungal and anti viral properties.

3. **Tea Tree Essential Oil** – It is great for your skin. It has many anti-viral and anti-fungal benefits, which make it the perfect preservative to use in skin care and hair care.
4. **Grapefruit Seed Extract** – It is an excellent preservative because of its anti fungal and anti viral properties.

A number of people falsely believe that synthetic chemicals are safe when you apply them to your skin. That's because they are sold to us based on hype and false promises, but the truth is that they are linked to tons of side effects and reactions. Some have caused a great deal of problems and in the very worst cases death before they are pulled off the market.

Mother Nature knows what's best for us, so it pays to try to live in harmony with nature, rather than trying to control it which almost always makes us pay dearly. Sadly, many of us will be diagnosed with a deadly form of cancer that could easily be linked to some of the skin care and cosmetic products we use. In the USA, 1 in 3 will be diagnosed with cancer. Avoid these chemicals and go natural. You'll stay healthier and you'll enjoy the many benefits associated with natural including a more youthful complexion.

10 Synthetic Preservatives to Avoid

These synthetic preservatives are chemicals and they are toxic. They often cause allergic reactions or more serious side effects.

1. Quarternium-15
2. Propyl, Methyl, Butyl
3. Methylisothiazolinone and Methylchloroisothiazolinone
4. Isothiazolinone
5. Imidiazolidinyl Urea (Germall 115) and Diazolidinyl Urea (Germall II)
6. Ethyl
7. Butylated Hydroxytoluene
8. Butylated Hydroxyanisole (BHA)
9. 3-diol, Bronopol
10. 2-Bromo-2-Nitro-Propane-1

This mix of synthetic chemicals is the majority of skin care products and cosmetic. These chemicals have been linked to the huge increase in cancer rates, which should alarm us, yet far too many of us still use these products. These preservatives have been shown to speed up the aging process exactly the opposite of what you are looking for.

Beauty Tip # 10 – Beeswax Benefits

Beeswax is a colorless liquid that the female worker bee secretes from her wax glands as she builds the honeycomb 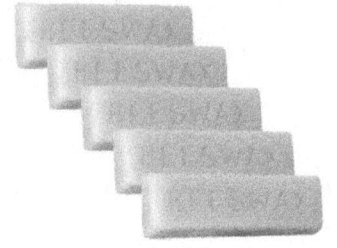 walls. Beeswax has non-allergenic properties making it useful as a skin protector. It is also an anti-inflammatory and an antioxidant.

Beeswax contains natural moisturizers that lock in moisture, nourishing your skin and keeping it firm. Beeswax heals the skin. Mix beeswax with other ingredients like olive oil to make lotions which are excellent for eczema.

The qualities of beeswax make it highly desirable in skin care especially in slowing down the aging process.

Beauty Tip # 11 – Essential Oils

Essential oils have been used way back in time to Caveman days. Today, essential oils still play a key role in natural skin care products and natural cosmetics. Not only do essential oils provide us with beautiful fragrances, they offer numerous health qualities, and they play a positive role in slowing the aging process leaving your skin healthy, glowing and more youthful.

When choosing essential oils make sure that you are choosing organic oils. Do not confuse cheap oils sold in department stores with therapeutic oils. Remember a couple of drops of pure essential oil go a long way. It should always be mixed with a carrier oil and never applied directly to your skin.

Let's have a look at some of the most common ones.

Lavender Essential Oil

Lavender is used in the treatment of acne, scars, oily skin, dermatitis and burns. It reduces the signs of age spots and regenerates skill cells so it's excellent for mature skin. Lavender can help you age beautifully.

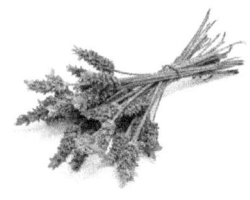

Carrot Seed Essential Oil

Carrot seed essential oil rejuvenates the skin at the cellular level so it is able to improve the tone of aging skin.

Orange Essential Oil

When orange is used in a lotion or cream it will help to detoxify 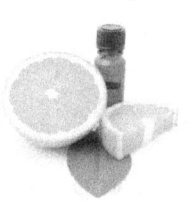 congested skin. It makes an excellent general skin tonic and works well for more mature skin, dermatitis, acne and to soothe dry skin. It supports collagen formation, which is necessary for healthy, younger looking skin and aging beautifully.

Frankincense Essential Oil

Frankincense essential oil has antibacterial and anti-inflammatory qualities that make it excellent for acne-prone skin. It is also a natural toner that will decrease the appearance of pores and even out skin-tone.

It protects existing cells and encourages new cell growth, which makes it useful in reducing fine lines and wrinkles, tightening the skin, and reducing the appearance of scars.

Ylang Ylang Essential Oil

Ylang ylang oil is extremely soothing and balancing for all skin types and it has a stimulating effect on the scalp, resulting in luxurious hair growth. Pamper yourself with ylang ylang skin care products.

Geranium Essential Oil

Geranium essential oil helps to regulate oil production and reduce acne breakouts. It improves skin elasticity and tightens 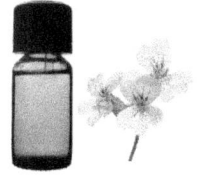 skin, reducing the appearance of fine lines and wrinkles. It promotes blood circulation to the areas where it is applied, to help broken capillaries, bruises, burns, dermatitis, cuts, eczema and other skin conditions.

Jasmine Essential Oil

Jasmine oil tones dry, greasy, irritated and sensitive skin, 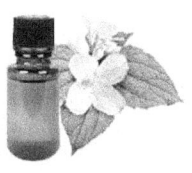 increases elasticity and reduce scarring. It is used in skin care products to improve elasticity and calm irritated skin. Jasmine is one of the most expensive oils because it is difficult to extract. Jasmine is picked at night when their aroma is most powerful.

It takes approx. 8 million handpicked jasmine blossoms to produce 1 kilogram of essential oil. Because jasmine is highly concentrated only a tiny amount is required in a product, which makes it affordable.

Lemon Oil Essential Oil

Lemon Oil is a natural astringent and antibacterial, so it is useful in clearing acne, removing dead skin cells, and cleaning greasy skin. Lemon oil can be used in a cream or lotion on the skin.

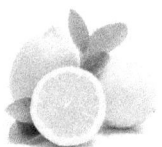

Tea Tree Essential Oil

Tea tree essential oil's antibacterial properties make this a good choice for acne-prone skin. It helps to regulate oil production, which can decrease the severity of your breakouts.

Patchouli Essential Oil

Patchouli essential oil is great for aging skin as it promotes new cell growth and smoothes the appearance of fine lines and wrinkles. It has antiseptic, antibacterial and antifungal properties, which can benefit skin conditions like dermatitis, eczema, acne and psoriasis.

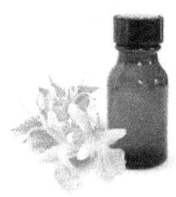

Neroli Essential Oil

Neroli essential oil is great for sensitive, oily and mature skin as it smoothes fine lines and tones sagging skin. Neroli is

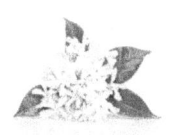

rejuvenating oil that contains citral, which helps regenerate cells. Its antiseptic properties balance oil production and shrink the appearance of pores without drying out the skin.

Myrrh Essential Oil

Myrrh essential oil is very beneficial to aging skin. It has strong anti-inflammatory properties that help improve your skin tone, firmness, and elasticity, while reducing the appearance of fine lines and wrinkles. Myrrh can also help heal sun damage, chapped skin and eczema.

Essential oils rejuvenate, restore, and improve the appearance of aging and wrinkled skin. Numerous studies have shown that essential oils can improve numerous skin conditions including acne, dry skin, eczema, freckles, clogged and pores.

Beauty Tip # 12 - Aloe Vera

The use of Aloe Vera in healing dates way back to the earliest of times. Aloe Vera has tons of healing properties and it can certainly help you age beautifully. Aloe Vera is one of the natural beauty secrets that is gaining a great deal of attention, with more natural Aloe skin care and beauty products coming to the market.

Aloe Vera can slow down inflammation. One cause of inflammation and aging is the formation of free radicals, which can cause wrinkles, and so Aloe Vera can be a powerful beauty agent, which is why it is used in many natural skin care products.

For cuts and burns, or acne, fresh Aloe Vera right from the plant works really well. There are also all the fabulous Aloe Vera moisturizing lotions and creams.

When Aloe is topically applied, it provides a protective layer on your skin, which evens your skin tone, reduces inflammation and reduces fine lines and wrinkles.

Beauty Tip # 13 – Make Your Own Skin Care Products

It can be frustrating trying to find natural beauty products that are safe and that work, not to mention time consuming. So many products on the market make claims they don't reach up to. It's exasperating.

One option is to make your own products. It's a lot simpler than you might think. A few clicks of your mouse and you may find all kinds of recipes online and we're giving you some that you can start to use right now.

Your skin will love it and reward you by looking radiant and more youthful. In addition, you'll be removing chemicals that your body no longer has to try to detox.

Let's have a look at the four main steps to skin care, and some homemade recipes that you can make right in your kitchen.

Cleansing Recipes

It all begins with cleansing. You need to be able to remove the dirt and grime. Of course, water is needed when you use your cleansers. Here are some excellent recipes for creating your own cleanser from all natural ingredients

Cocoa Butter Face Cleanser

Ingredients:

- 3 tbs cocoa butter
- 1 tbs Grapeseed oil
- 1 tbs water
- 2 drops sandalwood
- 1 tbs brown sugar with each wash

Instructions:

- In a microwave, melt the cocoa butter.
- Add in the water and Grapeseed oil.
- Whisk while adding the sandalwood.
- Store in a glass jar.
- Add brown sugar to your hands each time just before washing your face.

Lavender Facial Cleanser

Ingredients:

- 4 tbs Grapeseed oil

- 6 drops of lavender essential oil
- 1 drop of geranium essential oils
- 3 drops of rose essential oils

Instructions:

- Pour the Grapeseed oil into a clean, dark glass bottle.
- Add your essential oils.
- Gently shake to make sure the oils are blended before using.
- Apply a small amount to your face and massage into the skin. Rinse with warm water and a washcloth. Your skin is going to feel smooth and silky. This is an excellent anti-aging cleanser.
- Store in a cool place.

Dry Skin Honey Almond Facial Cleanser

Ingredients:

- 6 tsp almond oil
- 9 tbs whole milk
- 9 tsp honey

Instructions:

- Mix ingredients in a bowl.

- Apply to your skin using a circular motion for 1-2 minutes.
- Rinse with a warm cloth and water.

Oily Skin Honey Facial Cleanser

Ingredients:
- 9 tsp powdered skim milk
- 12 tsp honey
- 12 drops of apple vinegar

Instructions:
- Mix the ingredients in a bowl.
- Apply to your skin using a circular motion for 1-2 minutes.
- Rinse with a warm cloth and water.

Baking Soda Lemon Exfoliating Face Cleanser

Ingredients:
- Lemon juice
- 4 tbs baking soda

Instructions:
- In a small bowl, add 2tbs baking soda.

- Slowly add enough lemon juice to make a thin, loose paste. It's going to fizz and foam.
- Apply to your skin using a circular motion for 1-2 minutes.
- Rinse with a warm cloth and water.

Strawberry Acne Face Cleanser

Ingredients:

- 3 strawberries
- 9 tbs plain yogurt

Instructions:

- In a circular motion apply to your skin and continue for 1-2 minutes.
- Rinse with warm water. This is excellent for all skin types.

Moisturizing

Moisturizing your skin is very important, especially to help your skin age beautifully. When your skin is moisturized, the water is trapped in the skin, which keeps your skin hydrated. As a result, your skin looks plumper, less wrinkled and younger.

The Simple Skin Cream

If you want a hassle free way to make creams and balms without using preservatives here's a great step-by-step guide. There are only a few ingredients and it is simple and fast to put together. With no preservatives, it will have a shorter life span, so keep this in mind.

Ingredients:

- 6 parts Beeswax
- 3 part Almond Oil
- 30 drops Lavender Essential Oil

Instructions:

- Melt the beeswax in a double boiler.
- Mix ingredients.
- Pour into glass jars and let cool.
- Use morning and night.

Mature Skin Lotion

Ingredients:

- 4 1/2 oz Beeswax
- 13 oz Jojoba oil

- 18 drops myrrh
- 20 drops lavender
- 12 drops frankincense
- 8 drops carrot seed essential oil

Instructions:

- Melt ingredients together.
- Once melted blend thoroughly
- Let cool to about lukewarm, and then add essential oils.
- Cool completely.

Shea Butter Cream Recipe

Ingredients:

- 1 cup coconut oil
- 1 cup Shea butter
- ¼ cup almond oil
- 20 drops of your favorite essential oil

Instructions:

- Combine the coconut oil and Shea butter in a double boiler and melt on low-med heat.

- Once it is a liquid, add the almond oil and essential oil.
- Mix and store in glass jars in the refrigerator.

Anti Aging Wrinkle Face Serum

Ingredients:
- 12 tbs Extra virgin olive oil
- 30 drops of one of the following essential oils: frankincense, myrrh, rose, patchouli.

Instructions:
- Mix ingredients.
- Store in a glass bottle.
- Massage a small amount of the oil into your face and neck at bedtime.

Dry Skin Cream Recipe

Ingredients:
- 10 tbs of beeswax
- 2 cups of olive, almond, or coconut oil
- 2 cups of chamomile tea
- 6 Vitamin E capsules

Instructions:

- In a double boiler combine the beeswax, and a half of your chamomile tea, and your Vitamin E.
- Stir until completely melted
- Remove from heat and let cool for 10 minutes.
- In your blender, pour the remaining water and slowly add the oil mixture — it will begin to solidify and look creamy.
- Continue to blend.
- Scoop into glass containers – cover when cool.
- Store in refrigerator.
- Use daily.

Nourishing Facial Serum Recipe

Ingredients:

- 6 tbs Jojoba oil
- 16 drops Neroli essential oil
- 6 tsp Evening Primrose oil
- 20 drops Frankincense essential oil
- 10 drops Geranium essential oil
- 12 drops Carrot Seed essential oil

Instructions:

- Combine the ingredients in a dark glass bottle with a dropper.
- Shake for 2-3 minutes.
- Use 1 - 2 drops of serum over your face and neck.

Anti Aging Mango Butter Cream

Ingredients:

- 8 tbs Beeswax
- 6 tbs Mango butter
- 18 tbs Coconut oil
- 20 drops carrot seed essential oil

Instructions:

- Melt together wax and butter.
- Add the oil.
- Stir well, and allow to cool.
- Before the lotion sets add the essential oil.
- Mix completely until smooth.
- Pour into jar and let harden.

Exfoliating

Exfoliating is a very important in the care of your skin. It sloughs away dead skin cells, unclogs dirt/oil and leaves your skin glowing and healthy looking. Exfoliate no more than three times a week. Here's some recipes you can make.

Coffee Scrub

Combine 2 tablespoon of ground coffee with 2 tablespoon of water or olive oil. If you use olive oil, you don't need to apply the moisturizer afterward, as olive oil is an excellent moisturizer.

Baking Soda Scrub

Make a paste of just baking soda and water, gently rub it onto your skin and leave it on for 10-15 minutes before rinsing off.

Sugar Scrub Recipe

Combine 4 tsp sugar with 2 tsp honey and a squeeze of fresh lemon juice and mix well. Add more sugar if you find it is too loose.

Oatmeal Scrub Recipe

Oatmeal scrubs have been popular forever. It exfoliates and absorbs and removes dirt/impurities.

- Combine 2 tablespoon of ground oatmeal with 1/2 teaspoon of salt and 2 teaspoon of water or olive oil to make it into a paste.
- Gently rub it onto your skin in circular motions.
- Let sit for 15 minutes and then rinse.

Sugar n' Spice Face Scrub

Ingredients:
- 4 tbs ground oatmeal
- 4 tbs granulated sugar
- 4 tbs dark brown sugar
- 4 tsp cinnamon
- 4 tbs almond oil
- 4 tsp pure vanilla extract

Instructions:
- Combine all ingredients.
- Scrub your face with the mixture for 1-2 minutes then rinse.

Lemon Sugar Face Scrub

Ingredients:

- 1 cup lemon juice
- 6 tbs table salt
- Sugar

Instructions:

- Mix the ingredients and add sugar until the mixture is thick.
- Apply to damp face and let sit 3 minutes.
- Then scrub using gentle circular motions.
- Rinse well with warm water. Your skin will be smooth and so soft.

Sugar Facial Scrub Recipe

Ingredients:

- 2 tbs Milk
- Approx. 1 cup white sugar
- 1 tsp olive oil
- 2 tbs honey

Instructions:

- Mix all ingredients until it is a smooth consistency and not runny. Add more sugar if necessary.
- Apply to dry face in a circular motion.

- Wash off with warm water, then cold water pat dry.
- Store in the refrigerator.

Face Masks

A regular facial mask will draw out impurities and remove surface dirt and grime. Face masks are important in your anti aging treatments. Let's look at some easy to make at home face masks.

Rejuvenating Face Mask Recipe

Ingredients:
- 4 tbs olive oil
- 4 tbs milk
- 2 tbs carrot juice
- 6 tbs Yogurt

Instructions:
- Combine the ingredients.
- Apply to face, and allow to set for 15 minutes.
- Wash off with warm water.
- Great for moisturizing tired, dry skin.

Regenerative Wrinkle Face Mask Recipe

Ingredients:

- 8 tbs of natural green clay
- 8 drops of one of the following essential oils: lavender, frankincense, tea tree oil, or rosemary.
- Water

Instructions:

- Add enough water to make a paste.
- Apply evenly to your face and neck.
- Leave for 30 minutes and then rinse with cool water.
- Repeat 3 times a week.

Honey Face Mask Recipe

Ingredients:

- 2 eggs
- 6 tbs powdered milk
- 4 tbs honey

Instructions:

- Mix all ingredients well until they are smooth and creamy
- Apply evenly on your face.
- Let sit for 15 to 20 minutes.

- Rinse with lukewarm water, then cold water.

Apple Honey Face Mask Recipe

Ingredients:
- 1 medium size apple, grate finely
- 6 tbs honey

Instructions:
- Mix the grated apple and honey well.
- Smooth over the skin and let sit for 10 minutes.
- Rinse off with cool water.

Cucumber Facial Mask Recipe

Ingredients:
- 2 tbs instant nonfat dry milk
- 1/2 peeled cucumber
- 4 tsp plain yogurt

Instructions:
- Put all ingredients into a blender and mix well until smooth.
- Apply to your face, but avoid your eyes.
- Leave on for 15-20 minutes, then rinse off.

Avocado Honey Moisturizing Mask Recipe

Ingredients:

- 1 very ripe avocado
- 2 cups honey

Instructions:

- Mash avocado in honey with fork until smooth.
- Apply to your clean, dry face.
- Let sit for 10-15 minutes.
- Rinse well with warm water and pat dry.

Clay Face Mask Recipe for Normal Skin

Ingredients:

- 4 tbs green clay
- 2 egg yolks
- 4 teaspoon water
- 6 drops geranium essential oil

Instructions:

- Mix all ingredients and apply on face.
- After 20 minutes, wash your face with warm water.

Cucumber Yogurt Face Mask Recipe

Ingredients:

- 4 tbs brewer's yeast
- 4 tbs finely ground oatmeal
- 1 1/2 whole cucumber
- 6 tbs plain yogurt or sour cream
- 4 tsp honey

Instructions:

- Mix yeast and oats and set aside.
- Process the peeled cucumber.
- Mix in the yogurt and honey.
- Add the brewer's yeast and oats and process until smooth.
- To use, Apply to your face and leave on for 20 minutes, then rinse off.

There you have it – all kinds of great recipes that are easy to put together. Try one or all. Don't be afraid to experiment.

Beauty Tip # 14 – Eating Right

You've heard it many times - "You are what you eat" – when it comes to your overall health and well being and especially when it comes to aging beautifully this is very true.

 You've seen it with your own eyes. How do two people of the very same chronological age look so different – one can be youthful and look years younger than their actual age, while the other can look years older with a tired and worn out complexion.

Genetics certainly play a role, but one of the main contributing factors to how you age is what you eat. Your skin is your largest organ so it makes sense it can benefit from what you eat. Remember aging is more than skin deep.

It's all about the whole and unprocessed foods you eat, such as vegetables, fruits, meat, nuts, etc. along with making sure you are hydrated by drinking enough water. Drinking enough water is something most of us do not do well, yet it essential to aging beautifully.

As a modern day society we struggle with food and nutrition, our modern day society certainly struggles. Food allergies are on the rise, obesity is epidemic, people are not aging well - in fact, this is the first generation that will dye younger than their parents.

There are more chemicals and additives than ever before, being added our food. GMO have become a concern and that's just the one we are most aware of. You should be very concerned about what is in the prepackaged and convenient foods that you purchase, because they aren't real food and they will have a negative effect on your aging beautifully.

It seems that our generation has forgotten the importance of eating right and because of that many of us are aging poorly not just in our looks but physically as well. We gain weight and

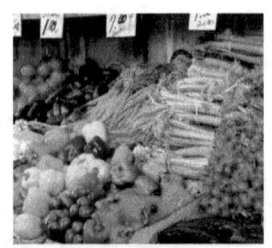

become overweight, we lose mobility, we have issues with our memory, we develop fine lines and wrinkles and we fight issues with our memory. We feel old – there's nothing beautiful about aging like this. Thankfully, it doesn't have to be like that. When you choose to eat healthy, get adequate exercise, and live a healthy lifestyle, aging beautifully will follow.

For millions of years, humans roamed the earth without having to worry about exposure to pesticides, chemical preservatives and processed foods. The diseases we deal with today didn't exist and they certainly didn't worry about again beautifully. That's because our ancestors lived a healthier life than we do today. We might have far more choices but they are not always good choices. Our ancestors ate to stay healthy and they aged gracefully. Not to worry, because we can change these things in our life. We can get our vitality and beauty back, both internally and externally.

You Are What You Eat

So what is a good place to start if you want to eat healthy and aging beautiful? Let's look at this in more depth.

Dermatologist Susan Taylor, MD, FAAD, is the assistant clinical professor of dermatology at the College of Physicians and Surgeons at Columbia University in New York, N.Y., and a clinical assistant professor of dermatology at the School of Medicine at the University of Pennsylvania in Philadelphia, Dr.

Taylor stresses that if you want healthy skin, to improve your overall health, and to age well a healthy unprocessed diet is necessary for.

The best way to make sure your skin and your organs are

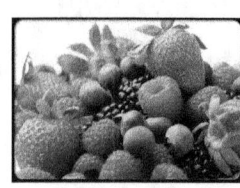 healthy is to make sure that your diet is healthy - optimum nutrition includes eating a healthy, well balanced diet. Your reward is aging slower and staying younger, more

youthful longer. When you are healthier inside and out, it's a win-win for you!

The Right Foods for More Youthful Skin

Having younger, healthier skin is within your reach. Research has shown that some of the best foods for healthy skin include the following:

- Beans
- Blueberries
- Fatty fish
- Green leafy vegetables
- Kale
- Lentils

- Mackerel
- Nuts
- Orange fruits, especially apricots
- Orange vegetables, especially carrots
- Peas
- Salmon
- Spinach
- Tomatoes
- Yellow fruit
- Yellow vegetables

Our ancestors were far more likely to hunt and grow the foods they ate. In fact, if we go back as far as the caveman, as much as 80% of the calories consumed came from plant based foods. Somewhere along the way, society changed, we grew less of our food and depended more on others for our food. With this came the loss of control over what we put in our body. You can get that control back by reading labels and making healthier choices.

We gave you a list of the healthiest foods for your skin and the overall health of your entire body. We should make sure that we have a diet that is rich in leafy green foods, berries, and nuts, because all of these are important to your health and play a major role in helping you to age gracefully.

Foods to Avoid

This probably won't surprise you! Processed foods of any sort, because they contain chemicals.

- Diets high in processed foods
- Refined carbohydrates
- Unhealthy fats
- Trans fats

You probably know at least one person that's over the age of 50 that is dealing with one or more health issues like diabetes or high blood pressure. Perhaps you know someone that is lacking energy. These people are not aging beautifully. They are not enjoying life as they age. If you could look at what they are eating it would reveal plenty.

Remember, it's not just about what we eat today but what we ate in the past. If your diet contains foods in one or more of these categories we encourage you to make some healthier choices if you want to age gracefully.

Diets rich in vitamins, minerals, and antioxidants will make you healthier and stronger. You will age well and you will enjoy longevity.

Vitamins and Minerals

It's inevitable - you are going to age – the question is not if you will age but rather how you will age. Will you age beautifully? Will you age gracefully? Will you continue to enjoy life as you age? Or .... Will you age poorly? Will gravity define you? Will it you deal with illness? Will you be limited?

All of us want to age beautifully, continue to be active and enjoy life. You need to make sure that your diet supports a healthy aging process. We talked about some key 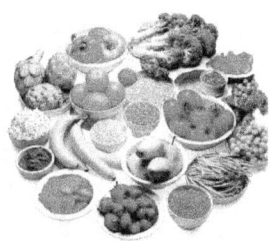 foods; now let's look at which vitamins and minerals you need to make sure are included in your diet.

Vitamin A

Found in egg yolks, oysters, and non-fat milk. Vitamin A depletion is often seen in those with cystic acne and is very important when there are skin issues.

Vitamin B

Found in red meat, fish, poultry, bananas, peanut butter, whole grains and eggs. Choose lean cuts of meat. Vitamin B is very important if you are suffering from skin issues. It is a powerful antioxidant. If you are fatigued your skin can become depleted of the necessary B vitamins

Vitamin C

Found in citrus fruits, cantaloupe, kiwi, tomatoes, sweet peppers, green peas and strawberries. Vitamin C is very important to those who are suffering from skin issues.

Vitamin E

Found in extra-lean meat, salmon, legumes, leafy vegetables, almonds, and olive oil. It is an antioxidant. If you are fatigued your skin can become depleted of the necessary Vitamin E.

Zinc

Found in turkey, pork, seafood, mushrooms and soybeans.

Selenium

Found in sesame seeds, tuna, whole grains, and wheat germ.

Essential Fatty Acids

Found in cold water fish, and flax seed. Essential fatty acids play an important role in the healing of your skin. They offer nutrients right at the cellular level that will reduce inflammation.

Making sure you are getting adequate fresh fruits and vegetables in your diet, along with low/fat free dairy products, whole grain pastas, nuts, seeds and beans. Avoid sugar - eat fresh…eat fresh… okay you get the message.

In a perfect world, getting the necessary vitamins and nutrients out of your diet would be easy, but it actually is not. Even if you make a real effort to eat healthy, we probably aren't doing it all the time and so you could be missing out on vitamins and minerals that you need to age gracefully and stay healthy. Take a natural vitamin supplement if you feel you may not be getting all of your vitamins and minerals daily. Read the label to make sure your supplements don't have fillers and additives.

Herbs

Since the earliest of civilization medicinal herbs have been used, especially as medication. After all, they didn't have doctors or to rely on when they were injured or sick. They knew the medicinal value of herbs and they created their own medicines to treat those who were sick or injured. Some of these herbs with medicinal properties are still used today and some of them are used in a variety of skin care products.

Aging beautifully includes taking care of all of your body, both internally and externally. It includes taking care of any health issues that come up and taking preventative measures so that you remain healthy to enjoy life. You can be active and healthy at the ripe old age of 80 – that's what you call aging beautifully! Aging beautifully is more than just having fewer wrinkles!

Water

Water has been necessary since the beginning of time. Nothing will hydrate you like water, and it plays a very important role in helping you to age beautifully.

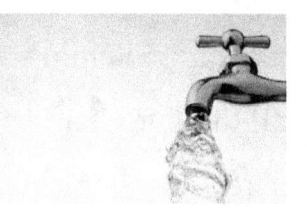

Women tend to spend hundreds if not thousands of dollars on all kinds of anti aging products with big claims. The sad fact is that you would be far better off if you simply increased the amount of water you drank and save your money.

Healthy skin begins internally. It doesn't have to cost you a small fortune and it doesn't require expensive products that are almost always filled with unhealthy chemicals. Your body needs its daily supply of water for you to be healthy and age well. Your skin needs water to stay young and supple.

Water transports nutrients you need throughout your body and it helps to remove toxins from your body, which can cause you to have skin problems including fine lines and wrinkles. Drinking too little water can cause you to be aged beyond your years.

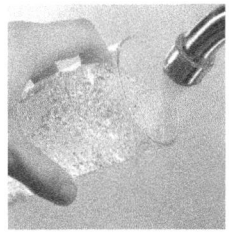 You need to drink at least 8 to 10 tall glasses of water every day. When you are working out you need to drink water continuously. Try to drink filtered water rather than tap water that has all kinds of chemicals in it.

Don't be fooled into thinking that bottled water is better because the plastic bottles it is stored in leach toxins. A better option is to invest in a good filter system that will remove the impurities from your tap water.

By consuming adequate amounts of water daily, your skin will be fully hydrated. Skin that is fully hydrated is fuller, has fewer fine lines and wrinkles and glows.

Don't forget that fresh fruits and vegetables are another excellent source of water. If you aren't drinking enough water you can make up the difference with fresh fruits and vegetables. When the weather is hot you need to increase the amount of water you drink by at least 25%.

Our modern day diet is packed with chemicals, preservatives, and toxins that your body cannot digest and that your organs are left to remove to keep you from becoming toxic. If the removal is slow, it can show up in skin conditions. Drinking adequate water will help you to remove the toxins faster.

Beauty Tip # 15 - Exercise

Diet and exercise are important and will help you age beautifully. We've already looked at your diet; now let's look at your exercise regime.

It's no secret exercise is good for you mentally and physically. To stay healthy and age gracefully, you need to ensure you incorporate exercise into your life. Yet most of us don't get nearly enough exercise. You can choose to ignore the fact that exercise is important, but your body will tell you otherwise. One day, when you look in the mirror you'll look older than your actual age. You will not age gracefully without exercise in your day to day life.

You might be paying out money for a gym membership, but are you using it or does it just look good on paper? For our ancestors being fitness was a necessity to staying alive, unlike today where we believe it is more of an option. The trouble is it isn't an option - it's key to staying healthy and aging beautifully.

Many are certainly not truly aware of the importance of regular exercise in maintaining healthy skin. We tend to spend our time focusing on cardio benefits not skin benefits. When was the last time you heard anyone say, "I've need to work out so my skin stays youthful." Chances are you have never heard anyone make such a statement. It's much more likely you would hear "I need to work out to keep my heart healthy."

When you exercise, it increases the blood flow to your skin, which in nourishes the skin cells and it remove waste and free radicals from your skin cells. That helps to keep your skin more youthful – the end result is you age beautifully.

The Right Work Out

There's no question that our ancestors were stronger and fitter than most of us are today. Fitness was really part of day to day life.

You don't need a trainer, nor do you need a gym to get fit. It's as simple as putting on your shoes and going for a walk. Enjoy all the many health benefits including slowing the aging process.

There are many workouts that are good – it's a matter of what your preference is. They can all help you get healthier and benefit your skin.

Aerobic Exercise

The goal is to walk 10,000 steps a day – that's what the experts recommend. A mile is made up of about 2,000 steps, and 10,000 steps is five miles. When you reach the goal of 10,000 steps, why not try for 20,000 steps a day.

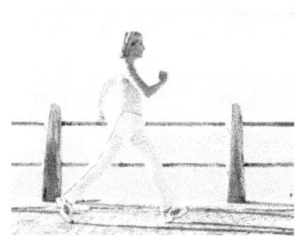

Power walking, jogging and riding a bike are few of the aerobic exercises you can do without any special equipment. There are tons of others!

Aerobic exercises increase the oxygen in your blood, which increases endorphin production. Aerobic exercise stimulates your immune system, and increases your stamina.

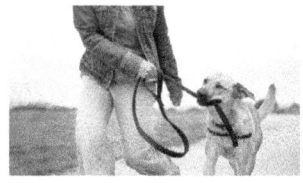

If you need a little motivational help, take your dog for a walk or ask a friend to go with you. Don't let the weather keep you indoors. If the weathers really ugly, head over to the mall and do a couple of laps. If the weather is too hot, go find a shaded park to walk around. Just do it – no excuses - just get moving. You'll be rewarded by staying stronger, aging slower, and looking and feeling more youthful.

Core Exercises

Another exercise strategy is to focus on your core strength. We don't often value a strong core like we should, but having a strong core reduces injuries, keeps us stronger, and it helps us to age more gracefully.

The trouble is most of us lead sedentary lives, and this has lead to a loss in core strength.

Your body has 29 core muscles, which are located mostly in your back, pelvis, and abdomen. This group of muscles provides the foundation for all of your body's movements.

When you keep your core strong, it helps to protect your back, improve your balance and stability, and make you less likely to injure yourself. Here are a few core exercises you can incorporate into your workouts.

Superman

- Lie on your stomach with your arms stretched out above your head.
- Raise your right arm and left leg as far off the ground as is comfortable for 5 seconds
- Repeat with your left arm and right leg.
- Do as many reps as you can reasonably manage.

The Plank

This is a great way to develop core strength, and you can customize it to fit your level of fitness.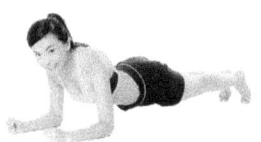

- Assume a prone position on the floor, supporting yourself on only your forearms and toes.
- Keep your back straight and your hips in line with your spine.
- Hold this position for as long as you can.
- Take a short rest and repeat 3-5 times.

- If you want to increase the level of difficulty, try adding leg lifts or arm lifts while you maintain the same position.

The Side Plank

- This is similar to the plank except instead of lying in a prone position, you are on your side. You will support yourself with either your left forearm and the outside of your left foot, or your right forearm and the outside of your right foot.
- Hold this pose for a long as possible.
- Repeat 3 to 5 times on each side.
- Be careful to keep your hips in line with your torso; don't let them drop towards the floor.
- You can also add arm and leg lifts to increase the degree of difficulty.

Oblique Twists with Produce

- Sit as if you were at the highest point of a sit up with your knees bent and feet flat on the floor.

- Place heavy round object in your hands and move from side to side, touching the object to the floor on each side. A melon works well.
- This exercise targets the oblique muscles and helps reduce those "love handles" that we all would like to see vanish.

Building a strong and stable core doesn't come overnight – it takes time, so be patient, because the benefits are worth it. You will feel better, have improved coordination, age more gracefully and look more youthful.

Strength Training

Adding just one strength training routine to your exercise program, it increases the benefits you get out of your regular exercise program. You need to tire out your muscles, and to do this you need to make sure you have enough repetitions.

For example, if you are lifting weights, you need to make sure you are lifting a weight that is heavy enough that you can do no more than 12 repetitions, yet light enough that you can do at least 4 repetitions. You need to rest your muscles for at least 2 days so that they can recover, repair and rebuild. That's why it's important to alternate the muscle groups you are working out.

Bodyweight exercises will help you develop strength, balance, flexibility, agility and coordination. The risk of injury doing bodyweight exercises is less than that with free weights or machines. With bodyweight exercises you can train anytime and anywhere.

To get you started, here are a few of the most basic bodyweight exercises that you can implement into your workout.

Push-ups

- Make sure you're using the proper form, or you won't get the desired result.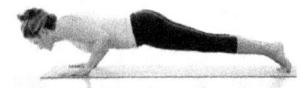
- To do an effective push up keep both of your hands below your shoulders and make sure they are pointed slightly outwards on the floor. Your hands need to be pointed straight ahead.

- Keep your back straight and lower yourself using your upper body weight.
- When you are just above the ground, push yourself back up to the starting position.
- In order for this exercise to be most effective, you need to do 10-15 pushups in a single session.
- If this exercise intimidates you a little, not to worry because are capable – push through it. Just start by doing as many as you can and increase every day. If that's one to begin with that's okay, because it's a start.

One-Legged Hamstring Bridge

- Lie down on your back. Make sure your body is straight.
- Extend one of the legs straight out while keeping the heel touching the ground.
- Using your other leg, you must push your entire body up from the floor, keep it in the air for 5 seconds and lower yourself back down.
- Repeat this exercise at least 6-8 times per session for each leg.

Burpees

- From a standing position, drop to the floor in a push-up position, kicking your legs out behind you.
- Do a push-up and then jump to your feet, jumping as high as you can.
- This whole body exercise strengthens your chest, shoulders, core muscles, and your quad and calf muscles.

Stretching

You need to remember to stretch before and after a workout. Stretching before you exercise loosens up all of your muscles, while stretching after your workout loosens up the muscles that have become tense from your workout.

Whatever exercise you choose, you should enjoy the effects of exercise. Initially, you may likely find you are tired after exercise, but don't worry, because in no time at all you are going to feel energized after your workout.

You'll enjoy all of the health benefits of exercise, including glowing, gorgeous, healthier skin. Exercising regularly will help you to age beautifully and stay youthful longer.

Making Time for Your Workout

The most common reason for not exercising is claiming to not be able to find the time for your workout. You are busy, you have tons of responsibility – we understand.

But ask yourself this – is my health important enough to make time? The answer is an emphatic yes!

You want to slow the aging process and look your very best as you age – keep your youthful glow.

The negative health effects of not exercising are significant, so do yourself a favor and recognize importance of exercise, so that you make time for it.

Here are five suggestions to help you achieve this. You got this!

Make Exercise Part of Your Routine

Research shows that even small amounts of exercise have positive benefits when you do them regularly over a long period of time. Park your car farther away than you normally would and walk to your destination. Use the stairs rather than the elevator. It may not seem like much, but it all plays a role in your health.

Rise 30 Minutes Earlier

It's not as hard to do as it might sound. Research shows that people who exercise early in the morning tend to be more consistent in their fitness routines than those who exercise later in the day. If you wait until later, there is a greater likelihood that something will interfere.

Wear a Pedometer

A pedometer provides you with great feedback. You might be surprised at just how far you walk in a day. Your pedometer will track your steps through your daily activities and this can really help to motivate you.

Incorporate Exercise into Your Leisure Activities

If you want to make sure you make exercise part of your daily routine, choose something you love to do. If you enjoy playing tennis or hiking, then incorporate those activities into your fitness plan. The more it seems like fun, the less it will feel like work, and then you are much more likely to do it regularly.

Ultimately, finding the time to exercise is a choice you will need to make. To enjoy the benefits you need to participate, not watch from the bleachers. By exercising, you will age more gracefully, stay more youthful and keep that glow. Isn't that worth the time it takes. You're worth it!

Fitness Tips to Remember

Now that you are ready to make exercise part of your daily routine, here are some tips to remember:

- Every time you exercise you need to warm up and cool down.
- You should exercise hard, but not constantly at your maximal effort.

- If you begin to feel dizzy, nauseous or lightheaded, stop for the day.
- Take a rest interval of approximately the same time as your exercise time during the workout.
- If you have health issues, you should always consult your doctor before you start an exercise regime or change your exercise regime.

None of us wants to age, but it's a fact of life, we are going to. 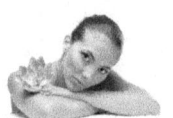 But why not slow the aging process and stay more youthful and energetic for longer, just by making exercise an important part of your day.

Final Thoughts on Aging Beautifully

There's no reason you should fear aging or wish could stop the process, yet for anyone 35+ it often slips into our mind – the fear that our natural beauty and youthfulness is going to disappear. By now you should realize that's simply not true. It's really a beautiful process. Your chronological age can increase, but you can still remain the youthful, energetic spirit you have always been. Be one of the women that become more beautiful as you age! Let's summarize.

- Avoid using skin care and personal care products that contain sodium lauryl sulphate, perfumes, and other chemicals. Instead, look for natural products that will provide you with healthier skin and no health risks.
- Avoid a diet that his high in processed foods that are likely to have chemical preservatives, instead opt for fresh, non processed foods. Make sure you are eating plenty of fresh fruits and vegetables. If you must eat processed foods or fast food be knowledgeable in what the food contains and make the best choice you can.
- Reduce your sugar intake. Sugar ages us and causes our skin to become dull. We lose that glow we long for.

- Drink at least 2 liters of water daily. Water hydrates your skin reducing the signs of fine lines and wrinkles and it gives your skin a healthy glow.
- Make sure you exercise regularly, and aim for 10,000 steps every day. Exercise will keep you young!

It pretty easy to grasp the benefits you will get from choosing natural skin care and cosmetics, eating a healthy diet, and exercising so that you age gracefully and maintain your youthfulness. But it might harder than you think to actually 'talk the talk' and 'walk the walk.'

We live in an age of convenience. When we want something, we want it right now. Our workplaces and our personal lives demand a lot from us –be fast, be smart, be efficient, pick up your feet and get busy, time is money, you're slowing production… and it goes on and on. We are all under a great deal of pressure to always perform optimally and thanks to technology that's possible.

Flash back to the days of our ancestors who had to provide everything they needed for themselves. Every day, they had to depend on their own abilities. There was no technology to rely on.

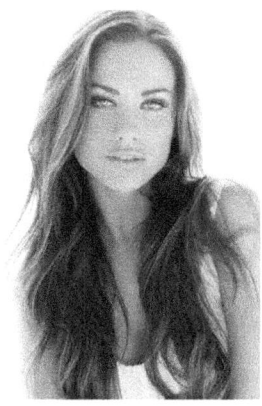

The life our ancestors was no easy ride—they worked very hard to survive. However, did you know that on average they worked only 4 to 5 hours a day, compared to our workaholic lifestyles of today? We could certainly learn something from our ancestors. Slow down!

It's the one thing we didn't talk about. It's quite possible that a simpler, more natural way of approaching our family, work, and leisure is a much better option. A simpler lifestyle can help to slow the aging process and keep us happier and healthier.

Yes, we know that this isn't always possible, but just keeping it in mind can help you to use your time wiser and make the most of your free time.

The choices we make define our way of life. Ultimately our decisions really are our own. We decide what time we will wake up, what foods we will eat, what music we will listen to, where we will work, when we will drive/walk, what we will do with our down time and all kinds of other preferences in our daily lives. In a nutshell this becomes our lifestyle – the way we choose to live.

There are also many external factors that affect our lifestyles – Social order, religion, culture, geographic locations, etc. – these are just a few of the exterior variables that play a role in our lives.

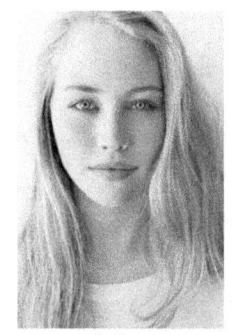 In the times of the caveman, a typical day would include hunting for food, socializing with other tribe members, caring for the children and elders of the tribe. While this may seem like a harsh lifestyle and one you certainly don't want to live, if we think about the materialistic world we live in, the truth is the lifestyle of early civilization may have been far healthier.

Our ancestors woke up only when their bodies were rested, not when the alarm clock said it was time to get up. They spent their days walking compared to sitting in traffic jams and trying not to lose control (road rage) over idiotic drivers. They worked from sunrise to early afternoon compared to our days that start early in the morning and end late at night.

What we tend to forget is that in general, even though we may not think so, we control our lifestyle choices – 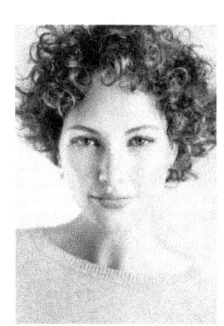 we decide what our life will look like. You might feel like you have no choice but to work a 10 or 12 hour day and live a life full of stress, but the truth is many times if you chose to live in a smaller home, drive an older car, go without some of today's luxuries, etc. you could live a different lifestyle. You have the ability to choose to the life you want to live and what's right for you.

When it comes to aging, your lifestyle choices can affect how poorly or how well you age. You can take back control of your life and live any lifestyle you choose to. You decide what's important to you. You decide to make aging gracefully your priority.

Everything we've talked about is easy to include in your day to day life if you want to. Nothing is extravagant or requires you to give up anything in your life today. It only requires you to make small changes and for those small changes you will reap huge benefits.

One Last Thought – It's All in Your Attitude

We want to leave you with one last thought – if you think you are old, you will be old – if you think you are young, you will

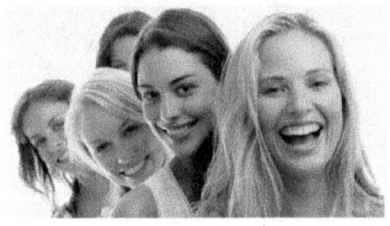 be young. How do you act? Have you brought along your youthful personality of years gone by.

It's all in your attitude, how you treat life, how you take life on. Ultimately, you will only be as old as you feel. Let your inner and outer beauty shine.

You too can age beautifully!

www.ingramcontent.com/pod-product-compliance
Lightning Source LLC
Chambersburg PA
CBHW071359310526
45790CB00019B/1553